New Edition!

The Lessons of Caring

Inspiration & Support for Family Caregivers

Santo D. Marabella, MBA, DSW

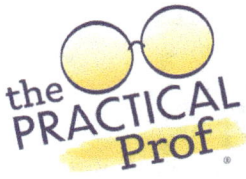

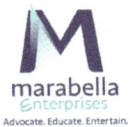

Copyright © 2024, 2019 by Santo D. Marabella

All rights reserved. This book or any portion thereof may not be reproduced or used in any manner whatsoever without the express written permission of the publisher except for the use of brief quotations in a book review.

Printed in the United States of America First Printing, 2024

ISBN 978-0-578-33786-9

Marabella Enterprises, LLC

www.MarabellaLLC.com

Contents

Introduction	V
Layout of the Book	XI
Dedication	XII
1. Lesson A The Losses are Many	1
2. Lesson B The Sadness is Gripping	5
3. Lesson C The Regrets are Avoidable	9
4. Lesson D The Role is Respect	13
5. Lesson E The Goal is Protection	17
6. Lesson F The Advocacy is Paramount	21
7. Lesson G The Job is Draining	26
8. Lesson H The Caring is Love	31
9. Lesson I After-Caring Cannot be an Afterthought	35

Author's Note	40
About the Author	42
Acknowledgements	44
Special Bonus	45

Introduction

NEW INTRODUCTION VIDEO to the 2024 EDITION

https://youtu.be/nN1Mq4g9YLw

I FIRST PUBLISHED THE Lessons of Caring as an e-book in 2018, then, in 2019 as a paperback. I am grateful to those who read it, and I've heard from many that it was encouraging and helpful, which makes me happy. A lot has happened since then. Enough to motivate me to publish a new edition and call it The Lessons of Caring... And Life After Caregiving.

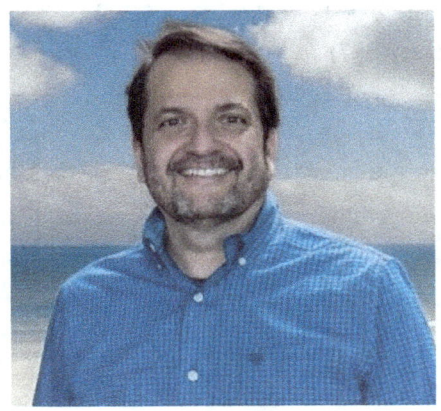

On June 29, 2019, my 89 year old Mom fell as she was reaching for some juice in the refrigerator to take her morning pills. I was on my way over at 6:15am to take her for her dialysis treatment. I always called to make sure she was getting ready and she didn't answer the phone. I know my Dad wouldn't answer, he couldn't get up by himself to get to the phone. I knew something was wrong.

When I got to the house, I found my Mom lying on the kitchen floor, conscious but her right ankle was in a position that no ankle should be – I knew it was broken and we were in for a trip to the hospital. Always concerned about her appearance, she agreed to go (not usual for her) but wanted to get up and get her housecoat and slippers. I told her I'd get them, that putting pressure on her ankle was probably not a good idea. The ambulance arrived. I explained to my Dad what was going on. And, off we went – she in the ambulance and me following behind in my car, not to dialysis but to the hospital.

I was about to enter a new phase of caregiving. Mom would be in the hospital and rehab for weeks at least, and Dad, cognitively sharp, could not take care of himself for more than a few hours at a time. Thankfully, we had an "angel" of a caregiver to help us as I was still working full-time at Moravian University. I never slept another night at my house. From that day forward, I essentially moved-back to my parents' house, the home I grew up in. And, while Raffi (my flat-coated retriever) and I would visit home for clothes and dog food, we never lived there again. But, we were together, so we were home.

Mom pulled through this injury – she had surgery and rehab and was home by late July. Once again, her feistiness paid off. But, her comeback was brief. Later that fall, we learned her biliary cancer returned with a vengeance – two years prior, they "thought they got it all" but didn't. The cancer was so destructive that it made dialysis treatments unbearable. Mom decided to stop her treatment. I clarified and probed, making sure she understood the ramifications two different times. "I know what it means," she replied sharply. "Okay, we'll do what you want." It was the hardest decision both of us made – hers because it would ultimately end her life, mine because I knew I had to respect her decision to end her life. I couldn't have imagined a more difficult scenario to play out for one of the Lessons I wrote about in the initial book. I had to practice what I preached, but it was devastatingly difficult [see Lesson D. The Role is Respect for more on the lesson; and, also Lesson H. the Caring is Love].

She was on hospice for three months, and lived sixteen days after she stopped dialysis. Mom passed as she lived - on her own terms. She left us on February 12, 2020, right before COVID. It was a beautiful gathering of friends and family, memorializing and celebrating my Mom's life.

Dad was lost – but Raffi and I, and our caregiver, Delia, got us all through it. We navigated through lock-down, being as careful as possible but also getting Dad out when and where it was safe. We made adjustments - like going to a restaurant around 3pm when it wasn't too busy for his big meal, and sitting in a corner away from any guests. His Parkinson's progressed, or should I say regressed. Everyday things – eating, sleeping, getting outside or in the car – became bigger challenges.

As his health continued to decline, I decided the best thing would be for me to sell my house and make the move to my parents' permanent. Once that happened and Dad saw that Raffi and I would be okay, I think Dad decided he could no longer keep up the fight. His decline lead to hospice, as it did for Mom. His last week was filled with songs and stories. I sang the songs to him, which he wrote, and he told me stories – some I had heard before, some I hadn't. It was sad and scary seeing his breathing so labored the last two nights. I called hospice frequently, not knowing how much morphine to administer and how often. Then, on Friday morning, May 21, 2021, at 95, Dad passed peacefully from complications due to Parkinson's Disease – as it is said, "you don't die from Parkinson's, you die with Parkinson's".

After Dad passed, Raffi and I got settled into our new routine. At the end of 2021, I retired from full-time teaching at Moravian (I still continue to teach part-time) to pursue theatre, film and TV projects I wanted to create and produce. In early 2022, I wrote, produced and directed, "The Caregiver" a sixteen minute short film. Not so coincidentally, I wanted to tell the story of the family caregiver, from their point of view. I want people to have a better understanding about what family caregivers go through so we can support them. It's the same reason I wrote this book the first time and why I want to publish a new edition.

Most of 2022 was un-eventful – no deaths made it a good year. Then came 2023. Raffi, by this time about 11 ½ years old, contracted trigeminal neuritis in June. It's a rare and debilitating condition that attacks muscles in the eyes, face and mouth. It caused corneal ulcers, no sensation in his face, and the inability to control his jaw muscles – in other words, he couldn't eat on his own. Thanks to great veterinary providers, we got him through the first round. Yes, there was a second. Apparently, it's not that rare when a patient gets it once to get it again. This time was much harder for Raffi to rebound. We did everything we could, but I was faced with those lessons again, the ones I mentioned above about respect and love.

After a comprehensive conversation with the vet hospital ER doc, it was clear that Raffi has no ability to help himself get better. So, I did what a caregiver has to do – put the being you are caring for first. It was excruciatingly painful to let him go. But, it was the only choice I had. Now, for the first time in my life, my "everyday family" was gone – Mom, Dad, Dog. The onslaught of grief was profound. I took some positive steps, but they weren't enough. I'll explain about that in the new lesson that has been added to this edition: Lesson I. After-Caregiving.

Besides the new lesson, I am adding a special bonus – a link that will grant you access to my short film, "The Caregiver. Simply click on the QR code or put the URL in your browser and you'll be able to screen the film. All of this is explained in the Special Bonus section (following my Author's Note).

I invite you to continue reading, as what I've reprinted from the original Introduction is still relevant and will give you the layout of the rest of the book.

INTRODUCTION to the FIRST EDITION

This book is written as a source of inspiration and support for the contemporary caregiver. *The Lessons of Caring* is short, sweet, and to the point – a relatively small number of colorful pages with video commentaries from caregivers to comfort you, and exercises and questions to help you. It's the book I would want to read for inspiration and support.

Additionally, here are a few notes about what to expect, or not to expect.

1. Though I'm an academic, this will not be an academic read. As with my previous book, The Practical Prof: Simple Lessons for Anyone Who Works (2014), this will offer accessible content and pragmatic, usable (you judge if it's "useful") advice.

2. It is largely based on my experience, not my research. I'm a single, adopted only child, of two Italian-American parents. So, what I have to share may have limited relevance and applicability to you and your situation.

3. I have no delusions that this book is an exhaustive or comprehensive presentation of The Lessons of Caring, it is merely the lessons I have learned.

4. The lessons are presented with a deliberate sequencing in mind, but they can be read in any order you choose. You may find it helpful to just read one chapter and then try to implement the "homework" in each lesson, rather than reading all of the lessons.

5. Know that your thoughts and feelings are justifiable, and that as each day brings new challenges – it's OKAY to slip and get frustrated. (Take this as a caring reminder, not a presumptuous intrusion.). Re-read a lesson whenever you need a "tune-up!"

6. Each lesson, including this Intro, has a short video clip. Watch it before, during or after you read the lesson – it's really up to you. You will hear other caregivers share their experiences as it relates to that particular lesson. (see the Special Note on the next page).

7. You will notice throughout this book, I talk about selfcare. It's as much a reminder for me, as it is a prompt for you. I'm still learning!

8. Finally, humor has always been a key coping strategy for me, and so it plays a key role in this book. At times, it may seem irreverent, but it's never meant to be disrespectful. Each lesson will end with A-Musing, a final thought about the lesson that you might also find humorous, or at least, something that adds levity.

I truly hope that reading this book will feed your spirit, recharge your energy and affirm your amazing and life-changing impact as a caregiver! It has been cathartic to write!

SPECIAL NOTE about the VIDEOS:

In the paperback and ebook versions of this book, you will have access to view the videos that accompany each lesson. Scan the QR code from your mobile device (i.e. smartphone) or click on the URL at the beginning of each Lesson, and it will take you to the video for that Lesson. It's that simple.

NEW to this EDITION

- Addition of a new lesson I. After-Caregiving (page 36)

- Addition of access to "The Caregiver" short film; access can be found in the Special Bonus section (page 45)

Layout of the Book

In the Introduction, I described some of the components of each "lesson" (or chapter). Below is the complete Lesson breakdown:

- The Video –commentary and advice from caregivers and professionals

- The Lesson – my experience and thoughts about the Lesson's topic

- A Mantra –a statement that when repeated, strengthens your resolve and your power

- The Questions –a question or two about the issues and challenges raised in the Lesson

- A Reflection –suggestions for thinking and considering the Lesson

- The Homework –activities to help you improve or work on the Lesson

- A-Musing – some levity to cap each Lesson

To Mom & Dad, who taught me how to care!
To Raffi, who took care of all of us, especially me!

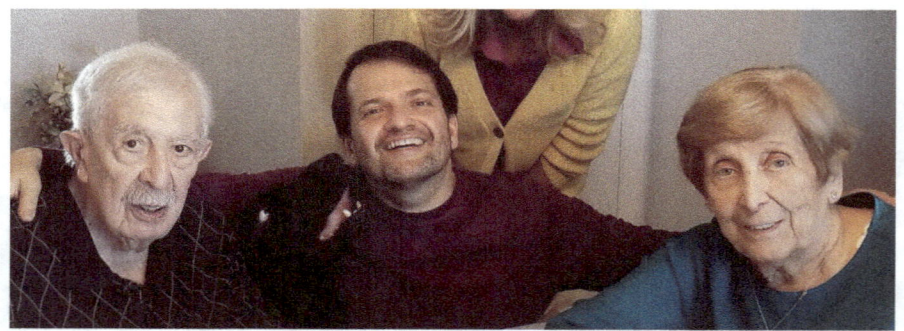

Mom, Dad, Raffi, and me

Lesson A

The Losses are Many

The Video: Losses

https://youtu.be/0zfNFTkCqJ0

The Lesson

"So take a look at me now, Oh there's just an empty space. And there's nothing left here to remind me, Just the memory of your face." (*Against All Odds*, Phil Collins, 1983)

My Dad, 92, continued to be an active musician for many years after he retired as a postal clerk. My Mom, 88, worked in hosiery mills and then as a hairdresser before she retired in her 60s. They have taken great care of each other and me, and still do today, as much as they can.

I never imagined how many and how endless would be the losses – I don't think they did either. First, there are the expected losses as one ages – the loss of friends and family, the loss of capacities and abilities and the loss of independence. As of this writing, my Dad has had Parkinson's Disease that was diagnosed 15 years ago, and my Mom is on dialysis to treat Chronic Kidney Disease brought on by uncontrolled diabetes. Each disease brings its own set of losses – physical, emotional and psychological. I was unprepared for the impact the losses would have on each parent and on me. I understood intellectually, but not emotionally or pragmatically. For example, the loss of my Dad's ability to drive made me THE driver. The impact on my parents is feeling dependent and guilty about having to rely on me. The impact on me is added responsibility and feeling guilty for not getting them out of the house enough. We're Italians – we excel at guilt!

In helping my parents deal with loss, I often forget to admit the effect that loss has on me, or I dismiss it as self-centered. Silly me, my Penn graduate social work education taught me, among other things, that I need to take care of myself before I can take care of anyone else. Don't think you're being selfish. Losses that our parents, spouses, siblings, children, etc. experience are our losses as well.

A Mantra

I acknowledge and grieve each loss, so that we (me as caregiver and you for whom I care) can move past loss and adapt to the new normal that emerges.

The Questions

Am I being honest about the losses that have or are occurring? Do I or they resent the losses? Are we willing to do the "work" (i.e. conversations, talk therapy) to get past the resentment?

A Reflection

Meditate, think, consider how loss is affecting your ability to be the kind of caregiver you want to be.

The Homework

1. Pick one of the losses that is creating tension or a problem.

2. Assess if it is impacting you (the caregiver), the cared for or both.

3. Decide how it would be best addressed: a casual conversation, a serious talk, an email or some other way. Remember, it may be that the best way is for you to "get over it," or come to terms with the situation on your own, as nothing else realistically can change.

4. Set a date (no more than 1 week) to address the loss, even if you are the only one it is impacting.

5. Address the loss – don't over think what you will say and do, or how it will go. Hold yourself accountable by having a trusted friend or colleague who you give permission to call you out, if necessary.

6. Reflect on how things went, what you would do differently or what you still need to do.

7. Celebrate the success – regardless of how small or large. Do something (e.g. go to a movie, have a meal with a friend, take a nap) for yourself – get used to hearing this, I'll be saying it often!

A-Musing

Sometimes as a caregiver I experience a "different" kind of loss – mostly, my car keys, cell phone, eyeglasses or Bluetooth® ear piece. There have been days when I've lost multiple items or experienced multiple episodes of losing things. Fortunately, I haven't lost my mind... although, close friends might say "that horse left the barn" long before I took on the role of caregiving – especially, when in one case at a lunch with a friend, I picked up her purse and belongings as I do for my Mom when we go to dialysis. But, what do they know – I never had a horse... or a barn!!!

Lesson B

The Sadness is Gripping

The Video: Sadness

https://youtu.be/MmZSE_RCcQQ

The Lesson

"When every little bit of hope is gone, Sad songs say so much." (*Sad Songs*, Elton John & Bernard JP Taupin, 1984)

Not surprising that with losses come sadness. At times, the sadness may be overbearing and all-consuming for your loved one, and perhaps for you. Often, it may manifest as anger, as it seems anger is an easier place to go to for many of us. I think this is because sadness is associated with being weak or depressed – and we don't want to be labeled as either. So we get angry, we get frustrated, we get belligerent – we get anything but sad, so we think. But, we're already sad, and the anger is just masking our sadness.

Blowing off steam, acting out our anger – this provides a good "release" of tension, but only in the short term because in this context it is not dealing with the cause of the anger – the sadness. When we address the sadness it helps to reduce our anger and heal our spirit.

One point of sadness for me, that I can easily become angry about, comes from the loss of my parents' support through their physical presence at artistic projects I have created. I can get mad that they're no longer able to attend my play opening, for instance. I can even be frustrated that they won't push themselves to "try harder" to be able to be there.

It does no good to be angry with them, and then with myself, for being angry with them. I'm not mad at them, I'm just really sad that my parents cannot be there for me as they have always been. It helps me to simply feel the sadness around the loss.

This acceptance of sadness is also helpful in dealing with their losses, or helping them deal with their losses. I have more than once (okay, like hundreds of times) reframed anger as sadness – theirs and mine. It has stopped me from saying and doing regrettable things.

But, first, I have to stop everything. I have to take The Prof Pause. What's that you say? The Prof Pause is the technique through which I immediately stop – I stop speaking, stop thinking, stop doing (all of which are very difficult for me). Once in the "state of Pause," I take a breath! Yes, oxygen is very important in this technique. Even with the very little I know about biochemical activities of the body, I do know that oxygen to the brain helps us minimize the chance of saying, thinking or doing something stupid. It's during this time that I'm able to reframe, reimagine or reperceive (whatever you want to call it), what looks like anger and see it as sadness. Then, I can be empathetic and understanding, rather than mad or frustrated.

Sadness, not anger, is your key to dealing with loss.

A Mantra

In embracing the sadness that accompanies loss, I find strength and perspective for healing.

The Questions

Am I blind to the sadness of loss? Can I see the sadness through the anger? Do I reframe anger as sadness? If not, what gets in the way of me doing that?

A Reflection

Meditate, think, consider how reframing sadness as a strength, rather than a weakness, can enhance your effectiveness as a caregiver.

The Homework

1. Think of the last time anger was present in your caregiving relationship.

2. Who was angry and why?

3. How well did you as a caregiver handle it?

4. If you would like to handle things differently next time, try this:

    a. When faced with an angry moment, invoke The Prof Pause.

    b. Reframe the anger as sadness.

    c. Empathize and understand the sadness. Ask questions or make statements like: "Are you upset about so many of your friends passing away?" Or, "It must be difficult seeing so many of your friends passing away."

    d. You may just need to let them vent and listen, not try to fix things, just listen.

A-Musing

There are times – more than a few – when I don't take my own advice... especially, when it comes to taking The Prof Pause. The times when as I'm speaking the words out loud, I'm saying to myself silently, "what are you doing? JUST SHUT UP!" By the time I've gotten to that point, it's usually too late and the "damage" has been done. I know the parents of some in my generation were known to wash their kids' mouth with soap for saying a bad word or sassing back. But, I need something else, more as a preventative measure... something like mouth masking tape. It would need to be flavored – cherry for me. I'll take a case of 50 rolls please!

Lesson C

The Regrets are Avoidable

The Video: Regrets

https://youtu.be/LVho4bAFjgM

The Lesson

"Regrets, I've had a few, But then, again, Too few to mention." (Paul Anka, *I Did It My Way*, 1967).

The commitments of caring – time, energy, responsibilities – can be numerous and onerous, but choosing not to care can be devastating on so many levels. The most crucial one to me is regret.

Before we address regret, we have to do some soul-searching about why we are caring. The best caregiving is authentic. By that I mean, it comes from a place of understanding our motivation for doing it. That's not an easy conversation to have with yourself, but the story you create will represent your authenticity. Here's how mine goes:

I was adopted by my parents as a baby. They gave me every-thing I needed and most of what I wanted. I have a wonderful life because of their love and care. I choose to care for them because of what they have done for me (paying it backward, so to speak). I also choose to care for them because I believe it is a beautiful way to "honor" them – that it's the "right" thing to do (I'm not religious, but I really get that 4th Commandment!). I also choose to take care of them so they have the best chance of having quality of life, for the life that remains. I am smart and resourceful, and can often help them have quality in their life. Finally, if I'm completely honest, a bit of me chooses to care because "karma is a bitch" that I don't want to mess with.

Understanding your authentic caregiving can help you avoid regret. Regret in my view is that ever-present, gnawing, underlying (or not so latent) feeling that "I should have…" Some regrets are more manage-able than others. "I should have stopped after my third slice of tomato pie (it's the lactose intolerant's savior)" is a regret I can get over! But, "I should have signed The Beatles back in 1962," is a regret from which Decca Records exec Dick Rowe probably never recovered.

In terms of caregiving, regrets are never something I want to experience. It isn't always convenient or easy, and it usually requires personal sacrifices. However, just the thought of not doing everything I can to take care of my parents, and having them pass, and then having to live in that reality would be torturous. Yes, I would be able to do the work to forgive myself and move forward, but why would I create that situation when I can avoid it. Avoidance isn't always a bad thing!

Therefore, I have made the conscious choice to use the threat of regret in my favor, when the commitment to caring feels overwhelming. Each time I feel this way, I remind myself how much I loathe unresolvable regret. It's not that I don't authentically want to care – I do; it's that in my humanness, I sometimes lose perspective. I know that it's a game I play, but unlike sports, it's a game I can win!

And, what do I win, you ask? The payoff is peace. Peace with my-self– no regrets means no guilt, and you know how much I value that. Plus, in the oft-times chaotic and unsettled world of caregiving, peace is a priceless prize.

A Mantra

I will choose to authentically care, because living without regrets will bring me peace.

The Questions

Do I understand my authenticity as it relates to caregiving? Do I live my life through a pattern of regrets? If so, is my caregiving important enough to me to break that cycle?

A Reflection

Meditate, think, consider how regret gets in the way of authentic care-giving or how having no regrets has freed you to care authentically.

The Homework

1. Search your soul honestly and identify your motivation for caring.

2. Create and write (yes, put it down on paper or in your computer) your authentic caring story. If you need help structuring it, follow this guide.

    a. First Sentence: a statement about you and your relationship to the person for whom you care.

    b. Subsequent Sentences: I choose to care because ___; include as many as you have, but at least three.

    c. Reread for authenticity – did I write honestly or did I only write what will make me "look good?"

    d. Ensure the balance – and add all the reasons why you are choosing to care; it's okay, you're not bad or wrong.

3. Once you have your authentic caring story, use it to help you avoid regrets. By being honest with yourself, choosing the "right thing" (whatever that is in your situation) becomes easier.

4. NOTE: You don't have to share this with anyone– it's yours. But, the benefits of doing this exercise will belong to everyone.

A-Musing

Regrets may be avoidable, but for me, guilt is not. Let's be honest – when you are a first generation Italian, raised Catholic, by Italians who are Catholic, the probability of avoiding guilt is negative 50%. Yes, I "hyperbolize" a bit, but my relationship with guilt is much like the way I feel about a day without sunshine– I can get through the day okay, but I'd rather have the sunshine! Guilt, while it does gnaw at your sense of perspective (and, perhaps, sanity),it also has amazing motivational powers. I'd like to think that when I teach students or speak to groups that I am motivating. Heck, I got nuttin' on guilt – it is the consummate "kick your butt in gear" tactic! I should market it as a new brand from The Practical Prof ®: Guilt is Good. Coming soon to a keynote near you!

Lesson D

The Role is Respect

The Video: Respect

https://youtu.be/Y5wKXvnjMVA

The Lesson

"R-E-S-P-E-C-T. Find out what it means to me." (*Respect*, Otis Redding, 1965)

I learned respect at a very early age. As a kid, I had to address my parents' friends as Mr. or Mrs., unless they requested otherwise (and many did, which is how I got a lot of "adopted" aunts and uncles). I was groomed to say "please" and "thank you," and to write thank you notes when appropriate. I was never to interrupt adults speaking, but to wait quietly until acknowledged. All of this taught me what it means to be respectful.

Respect took on a different form in caregiving. Now, it means honoring my parents' wishes for their life – including their health, their finances, their independence and their dignity.

Achieving this kind of respect requires a mastery of two equally important tasks: knowing what their wishes are, and keeping them distinct from my wishes. As for the latter, what Billy S said, "Ay, there's the rub!"

How do I understand their wishes? The easiest way would be to have an actual conversation about them. Wouldn't that be nice? Apparently, that happens in some families, but not mine. We talk a lot, just not about *that stuff*.

I remember a recent conversation with an old college friend about our parents. She relayed to me how she and her brothers sat down with their parents and actually had a conversation about their wishes, before there were crises or problems. I was shocked, and a teensy bit jealous. We have to have World War III to talk like that.

I have come to terms with the reality that I don't have it all served up for me on a platter – I just have to be a little more skillful in the way I pay attention and listen. Okay, a lot more skillful.

Here's an example. I open doors for people – men or women – including car doors. I just think it's being courteous and possibly I have a mini-campaign on "chivalry is not dead!" I've noticed in the past few years, that Mom prefers to open and close her own doors. How do I know? She tells me, "I can get it!" I'm quite perceptive that way. When she can't, she also tells me. And, then, I tell her to get her own door! No, I don't – I help her. The point is they do tell me their "wishes" just in bits and pieces, and they change as situations change. Listening and paying attention – that's how I know.

The other part of this is filtering out my "wishes." I wish my parents to live forever. They joke about that. They're realists, I'm less realistic.

Parkinson's has caused my Dad to fall many times, breaking many bones. Each time, he wants to fight to get back his mobility (albeit a little less with each fall), and each time, I'm there to fight with him. There will come a time that he won't want to fight. That's the time that I have to filter out my "wish" and respect his. It will be hard, but it will be the right thing.

I know their "wishes" could be self-destructive or harmful, but that's not usually the case. A book that helped me a lot with this is Dr. Atul Gawande's "Being Mortal: Medicine and What Matters in the End (Picdor, 2017). It may be helpful for you as well.

A Mantra

I will listen for understanding, without my filters no matter how well-intended, so I can honor your wishes and help you get what you need.

The Questions

Do I know her or his "wishes?" Do my "wishes" interfere with respecting their wishes? Am I good at listening and paying attention?

A Reflection

Meditate, think, consider how you respect the wishes of the person you care for, and if your own "wishes" muddle the way you care.

The Homework

1. Make a list of the "wishes" of the person you care for. If you don't know, find out by:

a. Asking them directly, or, if that's not possible,

　　b. Asking them the way The Prof tries to do, by paying close attention and listening.

2. Make a list of your "wishes" for the person you care for. If you're honest with yourself, you probably have a slightly different list.

3. Look for possible areas that your wishes might get in the way of their wishes.

4. Make their "wishes" the focus of your respect and help them make their wishes reality.

A-Musing

Besides what I mentioned above about learning respect growing up, "respect your elders" meant don't talk back. I've been told, by my elders, that I have a big mouth. It's not like I can put a tennis ball in it, but in the sense of saying what I think needs to be said, I suppose that I do. You may ask, "How does that work with the role of respect?" Not well! At least, not when one's big mouth is challenging a parent who you were raised to respect. Looking at the ingredients of every food product before it's put in the shopping cart and then vetoing it because it contains too much potassium; telling the doctor about a certain symptom that they "inadvertently" forgot to mention; calling the ambulance despite their protests that they don't need to go to the hospital even though they can't get out of bed. Big mouth – yep, GUILTY as charged! I told you I'm all about the guilt!

Lesson E

The Goal is Protection

The Video: Protection

https://youtu.be/U9x_J2y0ntU

The Lesson

"Demons'll charm you with a smile for awhile, But in time, Nothing can harm you, Not while I'm around." (*Not While I'm Around*, SWEENEY TODD, Stephen Sondheim, 1979)

I can't change the course of fate or life. I can't cure disease. I can't stop aging. The only thing I can do is protect my parents – specifically, protect their safety and their dignity. This has become the goal of my caring.

Sometimes protecting their safety is about their diseases and all the confounding elements they include. More than once during a hospitalization, I've had to question a healthcare worker about the medication they tried to administer which was wrong or the medication they forgot to administer. On one occasion, I overrode a doctor's order (not something I do lightly) and told the nurse to only give one-half of the dose to Dad. It was a new medicine and I was anxious about how his body might react to it. She obliged. Next day, the nurses called at 7am – they couldn't get my Dad to wake up. All his vitals were normal – it turned out he had a reaction to the medicine and was in a deep sleep for three days. And, that was with half the stipulated dose!

Other times, I have needed to protect them from themselves. I know this sounds like a contradiction to the last lesson, but you may understand with more explanation and examples. I've had to force them to go to the hospital when they don't want to go – my count is we're up to 7 times in 5 years, including one instance when ambulance, fire and police officials were at the house requiring Power of Attorney papers before they would take my Mom. She was septic and would have died had she not been admitted. Or, protecting their safety in the home, even when they think they don't need it.

One of the times both parents were in different hospitals at the same time (yes, it happened more than once), I had an alarm system installed, which I initially paid for. When I brought my Mom home a few days after Christmas, she noticed the bold security company sign in the front yard. "What's that?" she asked. "Your Christmas present!" I said. She groused a bit that day, but that was it. A few weeks later, she told me how she no longer "hears strange sounds" at night and has been sleeping better since the alarm was installed. I simply responded, "I'm glad, Mom!" PS. Not long after that, they insisted on reimbursing me for the expense of the alarm – I accepted!

Protecting their dignity is just as important. From helping Mom change her clothes in the ER with privacy, to going back to the dentist 5 times to get just the right fit so Dad can wear his dentures comfortably (I still don't think we got that one right!).

Lesson F

The Advocacy is Paramount

The Video: Advocacy

https://youtu.be/9EAbUcov9Ow

The Lesson

"*When you're weary, feeling small, When tears are in your eyes, I'll dry them all. I'm on your side.*" (*Bridge Over Troubled Water*, Paul Simon, 1970)

I could write an entire book on this topic, that's how important I think this lesson is. For now, a lesson will have to do. It is by far the most challenging and critical aspect for me as a caregiver. There are numerous, sometimes difficult, requirements for effectively advocating for your loved ones. I can say unequivocally that it is your strongest and most effective tactic in protecting those for whom you care.

It's not always clear what preserves their dignity, so I've learned to ask. Also, what's dignifying to me, might make them feel less dignified. Just because I don't think it's a "big deal" to be seen using a walker or cane, doesn't mean it's okay with them. Again, paying attention and listening is important to protecting them.

A Mantra

I will always protect you from harm that compromises your safety or erodes your dignity, even when you don't see the danger.

The Questions

Is my primary goal to protect them, if not, what is? What does my loved one need protection from? How do I protect them?

A Reflection

Meditate, think, consider if protecting your loved one is your primary goal, and how you achieve it.

The Homework

1. Identify one safety or dignity issue for the person you care for that is or may become a concern. Some possibilities are:

    a. Safety – falling, leaving the stove on, not taking their meds or taking them incorrectly.

    b. Dignity – feeling embarrassed, dependent, incompetent, disempowered or afraid of...

2. "Test" (i.e. ask, find out) if the person you care for agrees that they need protection from this; if they don't, assess (without your filter) if they

really do – be courageous about this!

3. If they do, outline what can you do, or what you won't be able to do, to protect them?

4. What obstacles lack of skill, ego, fear, etc. – may hinder your ability to protect them?

5. How do you plan to manage and ultimately overcome the obstacle(s)?

A-Musing

If I were a superhero, my name would be SuperSanto or ProtectingProf – I can't decide. One thing I know for sure is my motto. Ya know, like "…. and, who disguised as Clark Kent, mild-mannered reporter for a great metropolitan newspaper, fights a never-ending battle for truth, justice and the American way" (*The Adventures of Superman*, 1952-1958).

Well, mine would be a modified version of that. Something like: And, who disguised as Santo D. Marabella, a fumbling caregiver for great parents, fights a never-ending battle with healthcare providers, insurance companies, and anyone who stands in his way of achieving quality of life for his parents!

Lesson F

The Advocacy is Paramount

The Video: Advocacy

https://youtu.be/9EAbUcov9Ow

The Lesson

"When you're weary, feeling small, When tears are in your eyes, I'll dry them all. I'm on your side." (*Bridge Over Troubled Water*, Paul Simon, 1970)

I could write an entire book on this topic, that's how important I think this lesson is. For now, a lesson will have to do. It is by far the most challenging and critical aspect for me as a caregiver. There are numerous, sometimes difficult, requirements for effectively advocating for your loved ones. I can say unequivocally that it is your strongest and most effective tactic in protecting those for whom you care.

Here is my version of the requirements:

1. Be Proactive – depending on the scope of your authority and role, be the energy, catalyst, director and constant observer to anticipate next steps or new problems; I'm the power of attorney (PoA) for my parents' health and finances, if your scope is more limited, then be the proverbial "bug in the ear" of the person who does have the PoA; of course, always remembering what you've learned in prior lessons (i.e. respect, protect, etc.).

2. Do your Homework – read, call, email, meet with reputable sources (if you don't know which ones, ask one of the "experts"); sources include books, professional websites, media outlets, and people in the area that you need to advocate.

3. Pay Attention – to details, to subtleties, to what's not being said, to technical jargon that you have no clue of its meaning (then, do your homework and look it up or ask the "experts").

4. Go with your Gut – If you think something's not right, it probably isn't; if you've done your homework and you are paying attention, you will know when something's amiss or wrong.

5. Challenge the Experts – all and any doctors, healthcare providers, lawyers, insurance brokers and bankers. One way to help them understand is my "movie metaphor." The movie metaphor is this: the "expert" is seeing a "frame or one shot," but you've seen the entire "movie" to this point. They need to trust you to catch them up to the current "scene." You need to persuade them with your knowledge, insight, and charmingly engaging personality!

6. Find and Cultivate appropriate Allies – At the same time you are challenging, you also want to have credible allies who are inside and can help you navigate the system or obstacle; I have a first name, speed-dial

rapport with our hospital's patient advocate.

7. Be Relentless – they and the situation will try to wear you down, don't acquiesce; be firm, and be ready to escalate to the point of a hissy fit (haven't been able to ever use that term in my writing!) , if need be – sometimes it's the only thing that works (from my experience!)

8. Don't Take it Personally – words or behavior from the "experts" or the person you care for might sting, grow some coglioni (my Italian friends will get that!) and a tough skin; if you stay focused on your goal to protect, you'll be surprised what unpleasantries you can put up with.

9. Do all of This with Respect – for the most part, the people you deal with are competent and caring, but frequently, I have found some to be careless, and even lack empathy at times; so, while being respectful may mean you can't always be nice, as nice doesn't always work, you can always be respectful.

A Mantra

I will be an informed, proactive, and unrelenting "voice" for you, even when it means challenging status quo, systems, traditions and people.

The Questions

Do I have what it takes to be the advocate my loved one needs? At which requirement outlined above do I excel? Do I need more development?

A Reflection

Meditate, think, consider how advocacy has helped you or others care for your loved one.

The Homework

1. Pick one of the requirements I outlined above that you find most difficult to fulfill.

2. Through more reflection or a conversation with someone who knows you well, explore *why it is difficult* for you. For example, if #5, Challenge the Experts, is the one, you may find the answer in your relationship with authority. And, that may have developed out of your religious traditions or your upbringing.

3. Now that you have a better understanding of why, assess if this is work you can do or are willing to do.

4. If it's not, that's okay – your responsibility as a caregiver is then to find someone you (and your loved one) trust who can fulfill this requirement.

5. If this is something you choose to work on, consider this activity:

    a. Create a scenario similar to the difficult requirement; continuing with our example of Challenge the Experts, the medication the doc wants to prescribe for pain is a narcotic, but you know the person you care for gets confused with narcotics, even though they're technically not allergic to the medicine.

    b. Recruit a friend to play the doctor and you play, how about... yourself (good idea, right?).

    c. Tell your friend to be brutal – condescending, arrogant, emotionally disconnected (ya know, like a real doc... just kidding!); the role I'm creating for the doc is a composite of the worst providers, to help you the most with being able to challenge the experts. However, a significantly high percentage of the providers I have interacted with have truly been empathetic and helpful partners in my parents' health.

d. Practice the scenario for at least 10 minutes – painful I know, but it will be good prep should you encounter the real thing.

e. Ask your friend for candid feedback first. Listen carefully and respond to what they share. Try to be as open as you can. Then, share your assessment of how you did.

f. Repeat the practice component again, and give and take feedback as well.

A- Musing

If one more healthcare provider asks me if I'm a medical doctor, I may just have a full-out, terrible-twos, tantrum. And, to be clear, they're not being sarcastic, they actually think I might be a doctor or in the medical field, to which I reply, "I'm not a doctor but I play one in my role as caregiver." Okay, you can relax, I don't say that! What I do say is, "No, I just do my homework so I'm an informed advocate!" And, then I usually get the "look," the one that non-verbally tells me they're thinking, "oh shit, we've got one of those 'family advocates' to deal with," and I smile coquettishly without saying another word. The moral is: if they ask you if you're a doctor, you know you're on the right track as your loved one's advocate!

Lesson G

The Job is Draining

The Video: Draining

https://youtu.be/_2inEQnVp4s

Lesson

"*...EATEST LOVE OF all, Is easy to achieve. Learning to love yourself, It is the ...e of all."* (*The Greatest Love of All*, Linda Creed & Michael Masser,

...think about napping on the sofa, or at least continuing to type ...on. But, I am stronger... than.. zzzzZZZZZzzzzzzZZZZ. Oh, ...e 5 second power naps!

health.

    d. Practice the scenario for at least 10 minutes – painful I know, but it will be good prep should you encounter the real thing.

    e. Ask your friend for candid feedback first. Listen carefully and respond to what they share. Try to be as open as you can. Then, share your assessment of how you did.

    f. Repeat the practice component again, and give and take feedback as well.

A- Musing

If one more healthcare provider asks me if I'm a medical doctor, I may just have a full-out, terrible-twos, tantrum. And, to be clear, they're not being sarcastic, they actually think I might be a doctor or in the medical field, to which I reply, "I'm not a doctor but I play one in my role as caregiver." Okay, you can relax, I don't say that! What I do say is, "No, I just do my homework so I'm an informed advocate!" And, then I usually get the "look," the one that non-verbally tells me they're thinking, "oh shit, we've got one of those 'family advocates' to deal with," and I smile coquettishly without saying another word. The moral is: if they ask you if you're a doctor, you know you're on the right track as your loved one's advocate!

Lesson G

The Job is Draining

The Video: Draining

https://youtu.be/_2inEQnVp4s

The Lesson

"The greatest love of all, Is easy to achieve. Learning to love yourself, It is the greatest love of all." (The Greatest Love of All, Linda Creed & Michael Masser, 1977)

As I write this, I think about napping on the sofa, or at least continuing to type in a reclining position. But, I am stronger... than.. *zzzzZZZZZZzzzzzzZZZZ*. Oh, sorry! Gotta love those 5 second power naps!

A little tongue-in-cheek, but this caregiving gig can be exhausting. Some of the "drains" I experience are: worry, fear, lack of sleep, did I say worry?, physical, mental and emotional exhaustion, personal sacrifices of time and opportunities (social and professional), bruised ego or reputation, compromised ability to be empathetic (you can just get tired of being empathetic) and are you sure I said worry?

As you've probably noticed – I worry a lot. Caring for my parents has only exacerbated the neurosis that I've always battled. I need to work on it, but in the meantime, it's probably the greatest drain on me. I compare it to the old terror alert. I had been on Red (the highest level) for the longest time, but since our professional caregiver/aide has been full-time, my worry level is way down… to Orange (the second highest level).

I can probably blame worry for contributing to a "draining" evening for me, and four of our family's friends, in the ER. It was the same incident that I mentioned in the lesson about protection, when I had to force Mom to go to the hospital. By the time we got to the ER, I was a mess. I told them exactly what was wrong with her and why she was sick. I was worried the nurses would start trying to stick her to get the IV in (she's a hard stick), so I told them… firmly, "You can't go poking around – you get one shot and then call the IV team!" They did make a call, but it wasn't to the IV team. It was to Security. In less than a New York minute, we were escorted from where my Mom was to the waiting room. That's where they told me I was lucky we weren't removed from the property. Long story short, I was eventually allowed back in to see her – about 3.5 hours later. (Footnote: I was invited to sit on that hospital's patient advisory council so perhaps I wasn't such a threat!)

How do you know you're at the point of "drain?" Some clues might be: longing for a day to be sick in bed; yelling out loud at yourself, when no one is around, except the dog who starts to take it personally; being in a prolonged (more than a few hours) state of "pissed off"; and, my personal favorite, finding no humor…

in anything. That's when it's time to "repair the drain," or as it's more commonly known, self-care.

What works for me to "repair the drain" is a combination of things – living and inanimate. First is my dog, Rafaelle (you met him in the Introduction). He is a constant source of support and love that really recharges my energy and renews my spirit. (No, you can't have him – please get your own!). Then, there's humor. Humor is what my friend Carmela and I swear has gotten us through the most horrible, painful or difficult times, and I have certainly found humor to be a great tool to keep perspective as a caregiver. If I can't laugh or find the humor, it's really bad – and that's a big red flag for me! In that case, I pull out the solid go to's – our family friends. Sometimes I reach out to vent, other times to problem solve, or maybe just to share a meal together. Another thing I do is naps, just quick ones for an hour can boost my energy. Finally, and I don't mean finally as a last resort, I mean it as the last thing I'll mention in this list, is talk therapy. I have found talk therapy beneficial. Having an objective, professional perspective provide guidance in many aspects of my life, as well as caregiving, is a wonderful resource in my "toolbox."

If you pushed me to select just one thing that represents my greatest way to repair the drain, I would say unequivocally, it is having a channel for my creativity. I have always been involved with the arts, mostly the performing arts. As a kid, it was acting in school plays, but more recently, it has been as a writer (screen and plays), producer and director. I've realized that it's actually an extension of my teaching, just in a different form. When I write plays or for film/TV, I'm "teaching" through story. It's the same for anything I create – it's about growing and learning, myself included, in ways that are entertaining (I hope!). This book is the latest example of channeling my creativity. As I said at the beginning, it's as much for me as it is for you, the reader.

Oh, yeah, I sorta forgot one thing: physical exercise is probably something I should mention. Don't be like The Prof. He doesn't exercise. He knows he better start back at the gym. Be like the person who is disciplined with their physical activity so they can better manage their stress. Be better than The Prof!

A Mantra

I know that I must take care of myself before, and while, I take care of you. It is self-loving, not selfish; and, it is essential, not negotiable.

The Questions

What are the signs or cues that I am burning out or need to recharge and renew? Do I view self-care as selfish?

A Reflection

Meditate, think, consider how well you actually care for yourself.

The Homework

1. Select one self-caring thing that you don't do, but know you should do.

    a. I'll put myself on the hot-seat for this one and we'll use the example of exercising.

2. A little bit of change theory will help here. Identify the factors that drive, encourage or motivate you to do this – exercising.

    a. I can gain benefit from exercising for about 40 minutes, 3 days a week; when I actually do exercise, I sleep better, I can eat what I like without gaining weight, I have more energy, I'm less fatigued.

3. Good job, Prof! (encouraging yourself is very important!). Now, list the factors that stop, prevent, discourage you.

> a. I hate to sweat, I am embarrassed at how out of shape I am when I go to the gym, I don't have time, I don't like lifting weights, exercising is boring... should I go on?

At this point, you negotiate with yourself and see what negative factors you can change to positive, or how many positive factors outweigh the negative ones.

- Lifting weights is boring but maybe a fitness class with dance might not be.

OR,

- I live to eat. I can eat more of the things I like without feeling sluggish or putting on extra pounds when I exercise. I like eating more than I dislike exercising (not by much!).

A-Musing

So about exercising and that eight-part homework assignment I just outlined. Yeah, well, it doesn't work for me. I know it would be a great component of my drain repair. I know it would keep me centered and help manage my stress. I know I would sleep better. I know I could eat more of the things I like with less guilt (yes, I said less guilt!). I know if I actually did my own homework assignment, I would be able to break the bad habit that is such a wonderful source of guilt. My hope is that by calling myself out in such a dramatic way, exposing my vulnerabilities to you the reader, I will rise up to the challenge and do what is good for me, and restore some shred of dignity around this issue. NAAAAHHHH!!! Okay, I'll try, when I finish writing the book, if I'm not too tired, and...

Sometimes, we won't succeed at everything we attempt... and, that's okay!

Lesson H

The Caring is Love

The Video: Love

https://youtu.be/SyI711D5IRM

The Lesson

"ALL YOU NEED IS love, All you need is love. All you need is love, love, Love is all you need." (*All You Need is Love*, John Lennon & Paul McCartney, 1967)

I'm not a fan of most sports or crossword puzzles – my Dad is. However, in the past 4 years or so since my Dad has been hospitalized four times for months at a time, I've watched more sports and worked on more crosswords than I have in my entire life. And, I've really enjoyed it, well, most of it (except for the LA Times puzzle which is a lesson in futility for a novice like me!). Is it because I've suddenly developed an interest in either? Uh, no! It's because it's Dad-time and I have a big interest in that!

What I've learned the most about caring is that it is as much a gift to me as it is to those we care for. The gift is an opportunity to show and

feel love. How many kids get the chance to help teach their parents to walk... multiple times? I have been his coach, and he has defied medical science. A 2010 Annals of Internal Medicine, review of more than 40 years of studies, for example, found the risk of death in both men and women in the three months after a hip fracture to be between five and eight times higher. My Dad has had 2 hip fractures – both hips – since 2014. Even though the greater risk of death diminished two years after the fracture, mortality rates remained higher than those for older people who'd never broken a hip, even after 10 years of follow-up – and it was higher among men than women, according to that research. Maybe "love doesn't conquer all," but it sure makes a difference when you care for someone.

A Mantra

Caring for you is a gift of love that I cherish and appreciate.

The Questions

What gifts can I create through my caring? How will I perpetuate them?

A Reflection

Meditate, think, consider in what ways your experience with caring has been a gift – to you, the person you care for, others?

The Homework

1. Select one aspect of your caring that can be difficult to see as a "gift."

In the Lesson, I described two: watching sports and doing crossword puzzles.

   a. We'll take one of mine as an example: doing crossword puzzles.

2. Explore what makes it difficult to see as a "gift."

   a. As a teacher, I'm in my head a lot, thinking, so doing crossword puzzles seems a lot like work, rather than fun.

3. Next, look at the difficulty and see if there is a way to diffuse it or even transform it into something more pleasant.

   a. I find ways to make crossword puzzles less work and more fun: I cheat. I have my phone with me and when we've struggled with the last clue, or can't make progress in a "corner," I come to the rescue and look up the clue. It's amazing how many clues are "google-able!" (I'm usu- ally not proud to admit a flaw such as cheating, but in this case, I think it's rather clever!).

4. If that doesn't work (and trust me, with sports, sometimes it doesn't), then look carefully at the impact this aspect of caring is having on your loved one. There you will always see the "gift," in their eyes and in their heart.

A-Musing

As you read above, I'm not a sports nut –quite the opposite, I guess that would classify me as a "hater." Wow, that sounds harsh! But, it's probably true. I will spare you the psychoanalytic insight about why I am so pathetically "spiritual," but suffice it to say, that I don't have any skills playing any sports or any desire to watch sports. So, watching sports on TV with my Dad is interesting. I enjoy how passionate and knowledgeable he is about his teams, and I respect what a loyal fan he is to them. And, I genuinely feel bad or good, depending on how his team does at the end of the game.

When we watch games on TV, I am a quick study. Once I know which color his team is wearing that game – light or dark – I'm good to go. I understand the basics of most sports balls in baskets, balls in the outfield or in balls in the end zone – it's all about the balls. I can even feign disgust at a bad call by the ref or ump, "I can't believe that call! Wait til they show the instant replay, then, we'll see how bad that call was!" Speaking of instant replays, why do they even need a ref or ump? Couldn't they just have AI (artificial intelligence) review the footage and make the calls in real time? But, I digress… which is another way of "dealing" while watching sports! I'm a little bit better at watching sports in person, especially if it's in a box suite with unlimited food and adult beverages. Cuz then I can take my mind off the game and focus on important things like guilt from eating poorly!

Lesson 1

After-Caring Cannot be an Afterthought

The Video: After-Caring

https://youtu.be/FZSJyxCdsEM

The Lesson

"So I sing you to sleep, after the loving. I brush back the hair from your eyes. And the love on your face is so real that it makes me wanna cry." (*After the Lovin'*, Engelbert Humperdinck and Joel Diamond, 1976).

I was there when each of them passed away – Mon, Dad and Dog. When Mom passed, I had Dad and Raffi to take care of; when Dad passed, I still had Raffi to take care. But, when Raffi passed, I had no one to take care of... except myself. And, I didn't do that very well.

In mental health care, there is what's known as after-care. This is a form of out-patient care that continues treatment following a hospitalization. For the family caregiver, we need what I call "after-caring", it's how we take care of ourself after caregiving for our loved has ended. About a month after Raffi passed, I signed up to walk dogs at Humane PA. I figured I'd get my puppy-fix and help get some dogs adopted. I went weekly for two hours and walked and played with the well cared for sheltered dogs.

At the same time, I started talk therapy. I hadn't been going for a few years. No reason other than being busy and putting myself last. I felt that I needed an objective person to help me work through this onslaught of grief.

But it wasn't enough. I was consumed with sadness and grief.

I had no clue how powerful would be the impact of the grief I was feeling. I found myself in a very dark place. Confronted by poor choices and careless behavior, I knew I needed to make a change. I decided to begin the process of digging out of the hole I was in.

Lots more self-care began – grief group, reaching out friends, changing habits and planning for the next year, with the goal that it would be a better year. I decided then, when I took myself up to NYC over Christmas that I didn't want to be where I was emotionally. I know the only plausible (and desirable) way out for me was to look ahead.

I set three goals for 2024. First, I would coordinate a birthday party to honor Raffi's memory and raise money for the Humane PA Life-Saving Freedom Center – we raised about $2800. Next, I would put up a selection of my one act plays that had yet to be performed and give them a voice. They were well-received. Third, a project that is still very much in progress as I write this lesson, is the commitment to tell the story of my adoption with all of its beautiful and complex aspects. I chose a documentary film as I believe it is the most organic and engaging way to tell a story about adoption that explores loneliness, abandonment and belonging.

My point is – I didn't have a plan for Life After-Caregiving. This happened for two reasons. First, I didn't really have time to think about it, I was too busy taking care of parents and a senior dog. Second, I underestimated the power grief and delayed grief would have on me. I knew it would be sad, but it was immobilizing. I functioned (I always do) but it was a shell going though the motions without a heart. Getting back to a place where I could actually write about it took time, work, discipline and forming newer, healthier habits.

I don't want that for you. I don't want you to "wake up" to life after caregiving without at least some semblance of a plan. I want you to have peace of mind... and heart! That's what you deserve!

A Mantra

The present is the time to think of your FUTURE!

The Questions

What gifts that I have given in my caregiving for my loved one(s) can I re-gift to myself? List at least three that I will re-gift to me starting today, not in a selfish way but in a shared way.

A Reflection

Meditate, think, consider in what ways the loss of being a caregiver will impact you – social life, personal life, daily routine – all of these aspects are worth considering. If you haven't lost your loved one(s), it's still a good opportunity to fantasize what that might look like.

The Homework

1. Look at the person you are – as an individual person - in another role,

say professional or mother, spouse, etc, not related to your caregiver role. List the action or traits you deploy for that role. Now, look at your role as caregiver. List the traits or actions you undertake in this role.

   a. How different are the traits and actions" how similar are they?

   b. Are there any characteristics or traits from the caregiver side that you want to incorporate in your individual role or visa-versa?

2. Before we move forward, have you thought about how you will grieve the loss of your role as family caregiver? You may think that's it's a relief, or you may feel guilty that you didn't do enough. I hope that you honestly assess how much you did and how much your loved ones knew what you did.

3. Next, look at a vision of who you can and want to be in your life after caregiving;

   a. Do you want to fill that space and time with more from your personal or professional role?

   b. Do you want to take on a new hobby, class or skill, something that you've always wanted to do?

A-Musing

For me, dealing with this lesson in my life, I seemed to lose my ability albeit for a short time, to be a-mused. Except in very specific instances – the times I offered stories and anecdotes about my parents or Raffi during the events that celebrated their lives, I was able to find the humor. There were many situations that I was able to recount that brought levity – and the people who knew them could relate and enjoy the stories.

LESSON I

What I wish for you is that humor always is part of the most difficult and sad situations, not to mock or demean them, but to remind us that our flaws and imperfections bring levity and humor that can help carry us through. For some, losing our role as caregiver is a challenge to our future identity. Just as folks celebrate retirement from their jobs, we should celebrate the end of the caregiving chapter of our lives.

The one musing I will share is establish an exercise routine. After all these years, I finally discovered what gets me to exercise on a regular basis – it has to be social and it can't be competitive. Good luck with that you're saying, "right?" Well, I found three activities in the past year that keep me moving more physically than I've been in years. The activities are: pickle ball, aqua aerobics and dog-walking. I'll explain each one.

Dog walking. After Raffi passed, I decided that volunteering at the local humane society would be good for me and for the dogs. It has been good. I'm not ready to adopt a dog (not sure if I ever will be) but I get my puppy fix every time I play and walk the dogs when I volunteer, usually every week or so.

Pickle ball. I have never played a team sport – I was never picked (but that's a different book altogether). I was a bit leery about playing the game but pushed myself to learn the game. I have pretty much played once a week for the past year. I can say that I have made some progress – my skill level has gone from "horrible" to "not so terrible". Though there are still some individuals who won't play with me which is so seventh grade but whatever. I do enjoy playing with most of the people as they keep their competitiveness in check so I actually enjoy playing.

Finally, I have been going to aqua aerobics. It's usually me, two other guys and about twenty women. Needless to say it's very social and not at all competitive. And, surprisingly, I'm able to be chatty with the others and still get a good water workout in!

Author's Note

The Video: Closing

https://youtu.be/4QLVZklyDQM

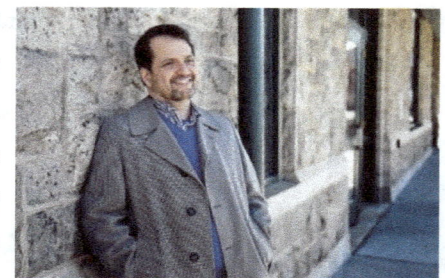

I began this book with my wish for you – that reading it would "feed your spirit, recharge your energy and affirm your amazing and life-changing impact as a caregiver!" I'm not that naïve (or arrogant, for that matter) to believe that one book – my book, to be specific would be able to do all that completely.

I do passionately believe, however, that when we reach out to others to share our lessons and offer our support – it does make a difference! It does lift us up! It becomes another positive tool, tactic or resource in our repertoire to be better than we are, and closer to the person we strive to be.

I want to especially thank the caregivers who shared their insights and experiences in this book. They truly are gifts to the people for whom they care. I appreciate your courage and generosity in contributing to this conversation!

Check out the video here. It will tell you how you can be engaged with this conversation and keep it going!

Thank you for reading. Thank you for caring!

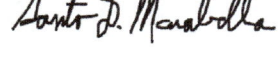

Santo D. Marabella

The Practical Prof ® July 2024

For More Information:

Author Dr. Santo D. Marabella, The Practical Prof ®, is also a speaker and trainer, focusing on topics that advance his philosophy to "manage with a heart, in ways that feed the spirit."

If you would like information about speaking, workshops and other special events, please email: Info@ThePracticalProf.com or click MarabellaLLC.com.

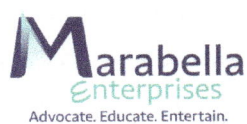

About the Author

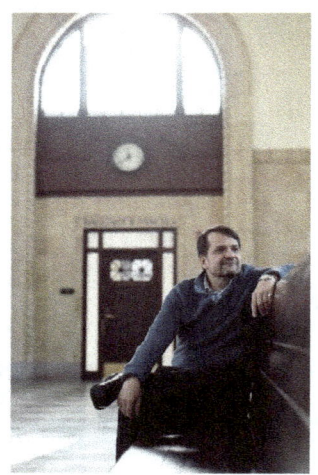

Dr. Santo D. Marabella
The Practical Prof® Author

Santo D. Marabella, MBA, DSW, The Practical Prof®, is an author, playwright, filmmaker, speaker and educator who creates, produces and distributes "Storytelling for Good". He is author of two books: "The Lessons of Caring," (2018) and, "The Practical Prof: Simple Lessons for Anyone Who Works," (2014) and his newspaper column, which has appeared in the *Reading Eagle's Business Weekly* since 2012. Marabella is a trainer/facilitator for the Greater Reading Chamber Alliance since 2015. He is writer and producer of an original musical (with songs written by his father, Sam), three short films and six plays; creator and writer of a TV pilot; producer of five short films and a TV pilot; and, director of more than 25 community theatre productions. He is most proud of serving as Producer of This Is Reading, and working with creator, Lynn Nottage, two-time Pulitzer prize-winning and Tony nominated playwright.

His current projects include a documentary film, "Il Mio Posto a Tavola (My Place at the Table) his adoption story which is being filmed in the U.S. and Italy, and, an original play of 5 one-acts called "Short Stage Stories: Rocky Road Ain't Always Sweet".

ABOUT THE AUTHOR

Dr. Marabella is Professor Emeritus of Management, Moravian University; President, Marabella Entertainment & Education Enterprises LLC; Co-Founder and former Film Commissioner, ReadingFilm; Co-Founder, ReadingFilmFEST; Co-Founder and Past Chair, Greater Reading Alliance of Community Theatres. His professional memberships include The Lambs®, the Dramatists Guild of America, the Academy of Management and the National Association of Social Workers. Dr. Marabella earned his DSW (Doctor of Social Work) from the University of Penn's School of Social Policy & Practice; an MBA from St. Joseph's University; and, a BS in Business Administration from Villanova University.

Marabella Enterprises Website: www.MarabellaLLC.com

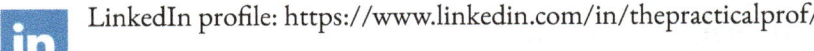 LinkedIn profile: https://www.linkedin.com/in/thepracticalprof/

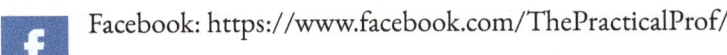 Facebook: https://www.facebook.com/ThePracticalProf/

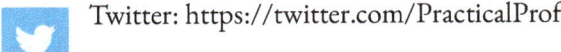 Twitter: https://twitter.com/PracticalProf

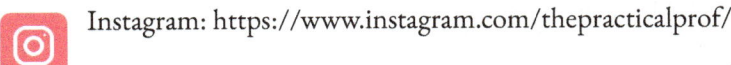 Instagram: https://www.instagram.com/thepracticalprof/

"Manage with a Heart, in ways that feed the Spirit!"

Dr. Santo D. Marabella, The Practical Prof®

Acknowledgements

Contributing Caregivers/Resources: Barry Ciabattoni, Sue Costa, Rev. James Lavoy, Kathleen Quartieri Swope, Lisa Pisarek, David M. Reedy, Kyle Ruffin, Rosemarie Sullivan, Barbara M. Thompson

Editorial Assistance: Kathleen Quartieri Swope

Video Editing: Andrew Pochan

Photo and Illustration Credits: Photo – Introduction, Santo D. Marabella: Moravian University Marketing & Communications; Photo – Rafaelle: Justen Patrick Lander; Photo – Closing: Natalie Kolb – courtesy of the Reading Eagle Company; Photo – About the Author: Lauren A. Little – courtesy of the Reading Eagle Company

Layout and Design: RH Publishing

Special Thanks: Marc Baron, for the idea to include the film with this edition; Michelle Hnath, for the suggestion to use QR codes before they were a "thing!"

SPECIAL BONUS

As MENTIONED IN THE Introduction, in addition to the new Lesson I. Life After Caring, your purchase of this 2024 edition entitles you to a special bonus: free access to the short film, "The Caregiver" (16 min runtime), written, produced and directed by The Lessons of Caring author, Santo D. Marabella.

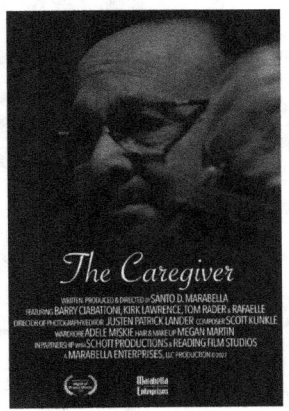

Accessing the Film

Simply point your phone camera to the QR Code and it will take you to my Vimeo site where you can watch the film for free. If you aren't able to access the film through the Code, then simply click on this link and it will take you to the same place.

https://vimeo.com/963718797/2febdc6eb0

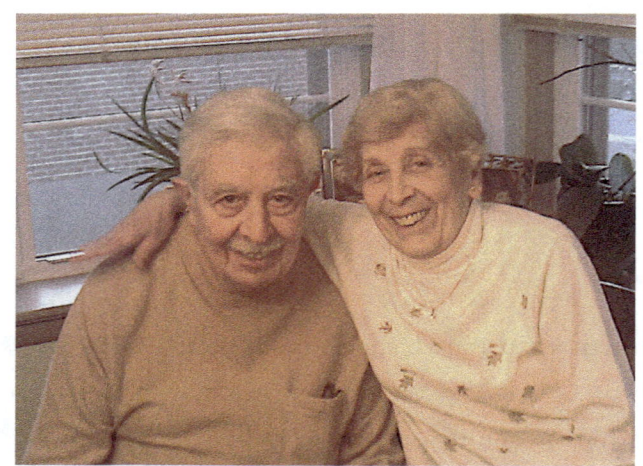

Mom & Dad, Thanksgiving 2008

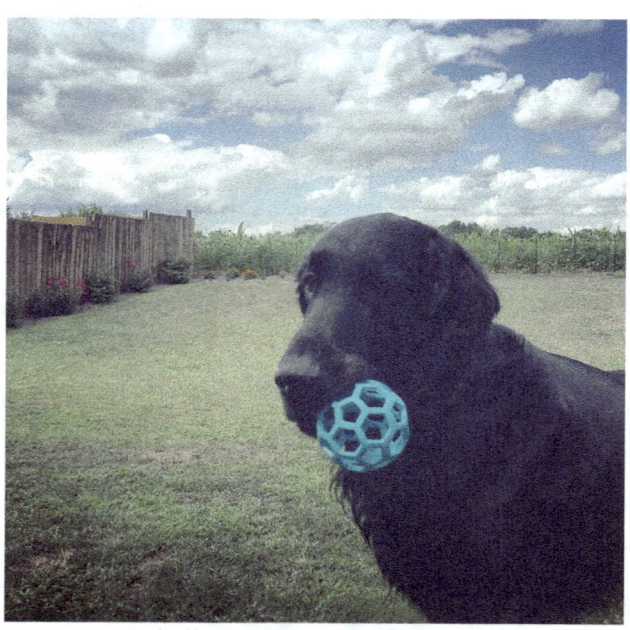

Rafaelle (Raffi) and his favorite ball

www.ingramcontent.com/pod-product-compliance
Lightning Source LLC
Chambersburg PA
CBHW071844290426
44109CB00017B/1918